Angels Don't Lie
Believe... Journal

Published by: Inspirit by Design, a division of Jeanne Street LLC, New Milford, Connecticut. Cover & interior design and illustrations by: Eileen Portelance New Milford, Ct.

Library of Congress Control Cataloging in Publication Data available on file.

PAPERBACK ISBN: 978-0-9974666-5-2

Second Edition, June 2020
Printed in the United States Of America

ANGELS
DON'T
LIE

Believe...

JOURNAL

Jeanne Street

illustrated by: Eileen Portelance

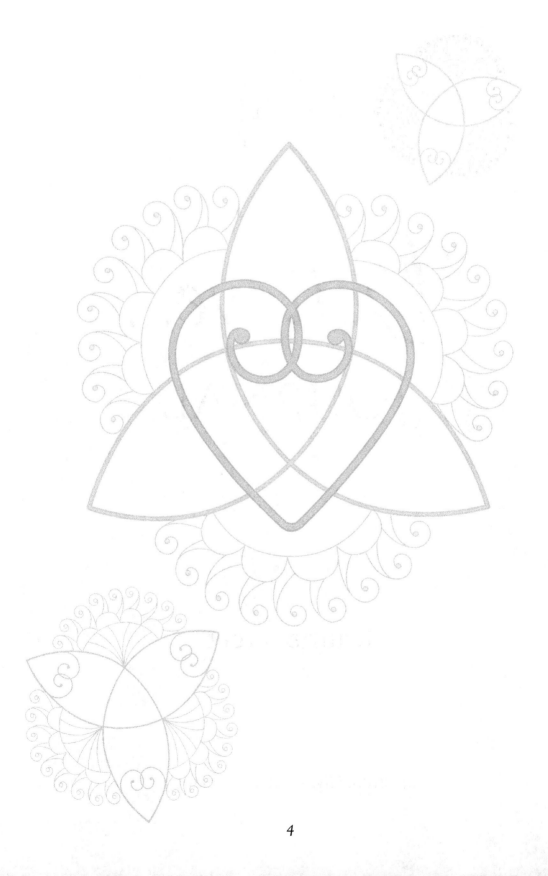

Dear One,

Within the journal you hold in your hands is a sacred space to express and witness your miraculous shifts. These pages are full of promise and supportive love for you. As you venture through the beautiful pages, you will engage with your inner wisdom and truth. You will expand your connection to the Divine and connect with your Angels. Calming energy will flow through your being as you work with the meditative prompts and release the words connected to your deepest feelings and hidden emotions.

You are a magical soul capable of connecting with God, Angels and the Divine realm. Through your deepened spiritual connection you can free yourself from energy that no longer serves you.

This is a companion journal to the book, **Believe...Angels Don't Lie.** I designed this journal with the intention of holding sacred space to support you in doing what I refer to as your "you work." This is the time and energy you spend on your well-being as you learn, heal, grow and evolve. Each chapter in this journal corresponds to a chapter in **Believe... Angels Don't Lie** and includes four journal prompts for you to free-write your thoughts, feelings and experiences.

Be at peace knowing your Angels will gently help to deepen your connection to Divine love and connect you with joy.

Before you begin each section take time to sit in a meditative state and do several rounds of cycle breathing. Then set your intention on connecting with the Divine realm.

blessings Xx, Jeanne

CHAPTER

ONE

ANGELS

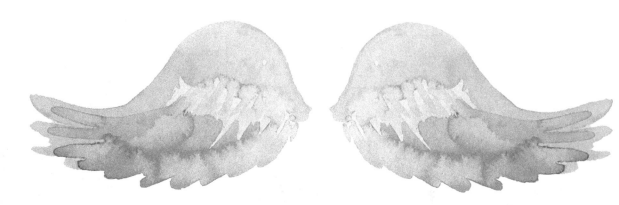

Angels are messengers from God. They can appear singularly or in groups. Their job is to gently guide and support you on your life's journey. Angels will never judge you or your choices. Their job is beautiful and simple: They gently guide and illuminate your path.

Fear is a feeling, an emotion, and an action. Fear can be felt internally as well as delivered to others. Fear tells you lies to keep you in a state of victimhood.

Living in a space of uncertainty blocks joy. When you feel doubt, when you're unsure of something you're feeling, or when you're pondering the truth of something you're reading, take a moment to call on the Angels, asking them to surround you with God's white light of love and protection.

How does it feel to be surrounded by Divine protective light?

$\mathcal{B}$elieve... JOURNAL

What do you notice about your doubts while surrounded by Divine love?

3

Asking for help is the first step to receiving. On the lines below, write down how, specifically, you need assistance.

Setting an intention is a deliberate choice. It is a contract you make with yourself to stay in alignment with love. Share how you intend to create sacred space for your "you work."

CHAPTER
TWO

KNOWING YOUR SOUL'S TRUTH

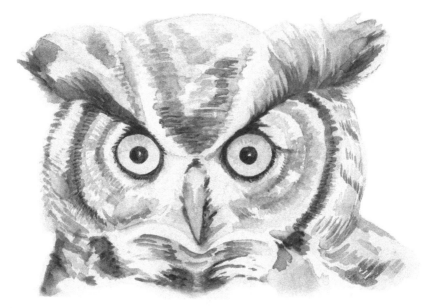

K **nowing your soul's truth comes from releasing old patterns, thoughts and actions that keep us in sameness.** The first step is to find your vulnerable side and expose the lower energy that isn't serving you. No one really wants to feel exposed. Yet when you stay in your vulnerability long enough, you will actually start to feel safe because you realize it isn't the situation that protects you; it's your own inner power. It is here in this uncertain and lonely moment of being exposed and uncomfortable that the authenticity of who you are can begin to shine brightly. Love embraces all of your brokenness. With faithful steadiness and security, love supports you to withstand any fearful moment.

Your thoughts turn into your reality. Your thoughts and actions are either healthy and love-based or they are low vibe and laced with fear. Doing the "you work" to be the love for yourself first will ultimately guide you to see where love has always been available to you throughout your life. No matter how painful the event, with enough "you work," you will find that love has always been available, and that you have been the one who has chosen to see pain in its place. Your choice to see love instead has the ability to change everything.

Meet me on the next page as you dive further into your vulnerability, this is your "you work".

Your relationships with others, and particularly the patterns within those relationships, can also show you the truth about your own self-limiting beliefs and judgmental tones. Your relationships are reflections of your soul's lessons. What are your relationships reflecting back to you?

Let's practice looking at your life with owl vision. Owl eyes will give you a 360-degree view of your past pains. Using this method to become a witness or spectator of your own suffering is a beautiful way of validating your feelings. It can help you to notice where love was available to you, as well as which lesson you can take away from the situation.

Reconsider a painful experience from your past and share what you can see by using owl vision.

After going through trauma, we experience grief. Both of these are powerful experiences that don't just go away with time. Instead, a new normal welcomes itself into our life.

Write about a grief you are carrying and ask yourself: Are you a victim coming from the standpoint of "I am grief" or an empowered being who is experiencing grief and who understands, "I have grief"?

Your outer world reflects the energetic state of your inner being. First, write in detail about how your body feels. Then, explain how your home and work surroundings mirror that feeling for you.

CHAPTER THREE

DIVINE CHRIST ENERGY

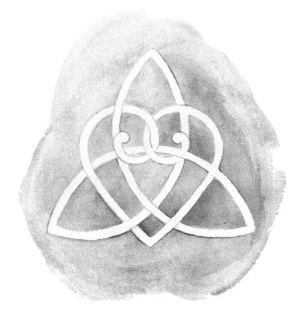

In my meditation, Jesus taught me the three holy Christ points. The hands are the first point, the feet are the second, and the heart and lung area are the third. The three Christ points are connection points or, as some call them, chakra points. Working with your Christ points is similar to working with your chakra energy centers. You open these centers by inviting the Divine in through prayer, intent, and angelic guidance. Then the energy will open, balance, and flow through your being. Your palms and the soles of your feet often start to tingle slightly, and then you may feel warm vibrating energy flowing outward.

God says, "Pray unto Me, through My Son, the Holy Spirit, Angels and archangels, and I will answer so you may find peace comfort and guidance. Pray unto Me, your weaknesses, and I will make you whole. Pray unto Me, your sins, and you shall be set free. In all things see Me and in all things, I see you. Blessed be all who rejoice in the Glory of God."

There are no perfect prayers or a right way of talking to God. He is always available to listen and hear our heart's desires, questions and petitions at any given moment.

Before journaling take a moment to say a prayer of petition aligning with the Divine and opening your Christ points. Now you can go forward to the journal prompts and connect with the Archangels..

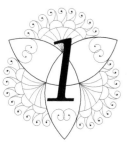

Archangel Michael will protect you with the sword of God's love while shielding you from the darkness, allowing Divine light to touch you.

First, close your eyes and invite Archangel Michael into this moment, gently asking for what you need with pure intention and love, and have faith that your needs will be met. Then, share your petition and experience with Archangel Michael.

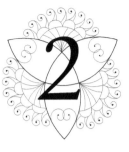

Archangel Gabriel is a loyal messenger, eager to deliver truth with kindness, gentleness and ease. Archangel Gabriel's loyal yellow tone and loving nature will empower your ability to speak truth.

Call upon Archangel Gabriel on the lines below to aid you in softening an area of your life. Share a petition for Archangel Gabriel to deliver for you.

Archangel Raphael exudes knowledge of many subjects and matters dealing with the well-being of the human condition. Tried-and-true Archangel Raphael will bear witness to your pain and suffering to better guide you toward love's light and healing.

First, outline an area in need of healing on the lines below. Then, invite Archangel Raphael to witness your pain and assist you on your journey to well-being.

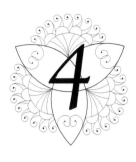

Archangel Uriel takes the form wisdom would take if wisdom were a man. He carries with him knowledge and kindness of God's will. Archangel Uriel will help you sort out the parts of your thought system that are based on fearful, lower energy and help you to realign with God's truth.

Write down the higher wisdom or the justice you seek and invite Archangel Uriel to swiftly guide you with the all-knowing truth of God's will.

CHAPTER FOUR

YOUR HIGHEST GOOD

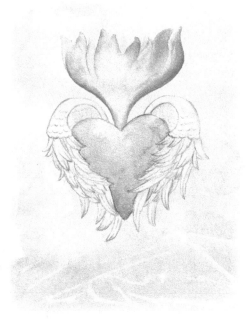

Your heart reveals the core of who you are. The Divine knows this truth and is always guiding you to experience challenges that form the essence of your life. This is because God is intent on building your character.

Choosing your path is your soul's destiny; you can align with truth or with fear. In any given moment you can choose to go it alone, follow fear or to choose love, and in choosing love you choose God. God wants you to live with love, abundance, and joy. These are all readily available for you when you choose them. When you put into perspective that your life's lessons, pain, and suffering are the challenges your soul must go through in order to remember, grow, and remain connected to God and Divine love, you can better understand that your purpose is to be the love your soul is seeking.

Angels are guiding you even when you are not aware of it. Gently, without force, they bring things to your awareness that will serve your highest good. Books, music, art, cooking, classes, people—the list of ways the Divine will gift you energy to propel you forward in your alignment is endless.

You have been gifted free will. Choosing your path is your soul's destiny; you can align with truth or with fear. In any given moment, you can choose either to follow fear and go it alone or to choose love.

Share how God wants you to live with love, abundance and joy on the lines below.

Your soul is here to be challenged, to learn valuable lessons and to expand from these moments.

Write out the current challenges you are facing and what lesson you feel is showing up at this time.

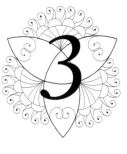

Love is the first thing you learn to forget. You were born with pure love, but it began to fade through your exposure to other viewpoints from your family, friends, and others. Their fears slip in and begin to manipulate your thoughts.

Describe the conditioned view points you were taught early on that don't resonate with your soul's truths.

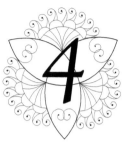

When you see or feel someone's fear, you can inadvertently take that fear on without being aware of it. You then begin to react to that sponged-up fear. All of a sudden, without warning, your reactions are bigger than you are. Your feelings and emotions get conjumbled up.

Think of a time when you felt someone else's fears. How did you feel? How did you react?

_____

_____

_____

_____

_____

_____

_____

_____

_____

_____

_____

_____

_____

_____

_____

_____

_____

_____

_____

_____

_____

_____

_____

_____

_____

_____

_____

_____

_____

_____

_____

_____

_____

_____

_____

Chapter Five

OUR LIFE PATH

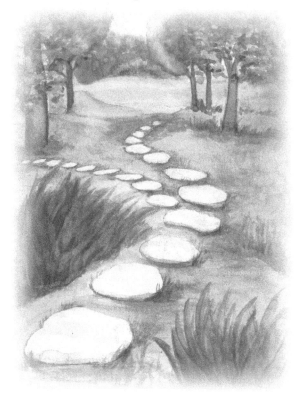

God does have a plan for you, it is intertwined with the path you have chosen to experience in this life. God also says that you are an invaluable soul with endless choices to make. It's up to you to fulfill the reason you have been born. Your reason is unique to you; your lessons, value system, and choices are all yours.

The Angels say that your destined life can have many outcomes, not just one path. Destiny is predesigned, yet not written in stone because you have been gifted free will to choose. While bad things do happen to good people, good people also make mistakes. It's just a matter of removing fear to see the truth. Lessons that challenge you can be the stopping point of your life or the pathway for your greatest growth.

Although everyone's life experience will be different, your soul's lessons will repeat until they are healed. Lessons can seem painful, annoying, and downright senseless, but they are your soul's pathway to enlightenment. Enlightenment is achieved when your soul has healed from the pain learned through your lessons and when you live life purely in alignment with God

Collectively, souls will also come together in life to experience lessons on a larger level.

Write down the lineage of lessons that have been passed down or are currently present in your life.

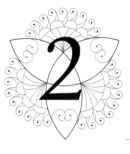

"Depression comes from living in the past, anxiety comes from living in the future, but love is in the present." This means love is your gift of being in this moment—but sometimes, it can be hard to see that.

Share your experiences with depression and or anxiety.

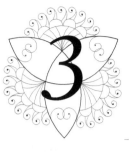

Your soul is infinite, so experiences and people come into your life to support your soul's journey. Although they may challenge you, hurt or anger you, they are here to teach you.

What relationships challenge you the most? What do you feel they are trying to teach you?

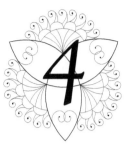

You can send your love, compassion and forgiveness outward to the one who caused you pain. When you allow yourself to see them as your equal or as your teacher, you are able to free your energy and theirs from being bound to the past.

Who can you set free, and how can you do so?

CHAPTER SIX

THE PERSONAL MORAL CODE

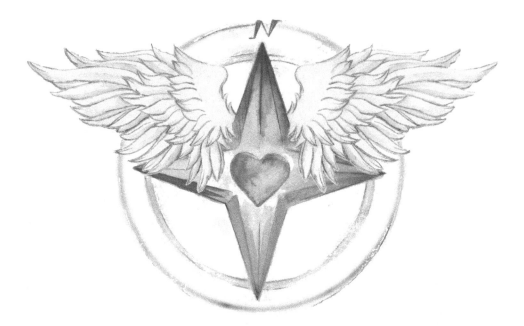

You have a personal moral code, or PMC, by which to live. The PMC is your soul's contract with God to live a love-based life wherein you dedicate yourself to learning specific and unique lessons. The PMC of your soul is designed by God and is woven into your soul's journey.

When your PMC is off, your choices go against love, and your soul's lessons become burdens that you struggle to carry instead of opportunities for learning and growth.

The Angels want you to know that fear is the most common reason that your pain and suffering remains unhealed. You end up holding these memories in your body, which act as a type of storage unit for old, unprocessed fear. While it is true that you will hold loving memories inside your bodies as well, they are not harmful; their energy is light, bright, and airy. These loving memories remain part of your memory center and connect with your heart. This is why when you think of a happy memory, your brain triggers a response and sends a signal for your heart to open. You feel lighter and brighter.

Hold yourself in compassion and love as you move through the next four journal prompts.

1

We all have at least one main life lesson that we've come here to learn. What do you feel or think your main life lesson is?

Look back over your past relationships and notice the common themes between them, as well as any similarities to your present relationships. Then, write them down. What are these themes trying to teach you?

3

Sometimes, these themes group together to form a clear pattern that is repeated over and over. Do you have a pattern of repeating relationships with people? What is the pattern?

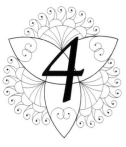

Fear energy draws you in, enticing you with false hope of something gained. When you give in to this false hope, you end up losing valuable time that your soul needs to experience and expand in this life. This inevitably transforms into a fear-based addiction.

Where is fear holding you in a state of sameness?

Chapter Seven

GIFTS AND TALENTS

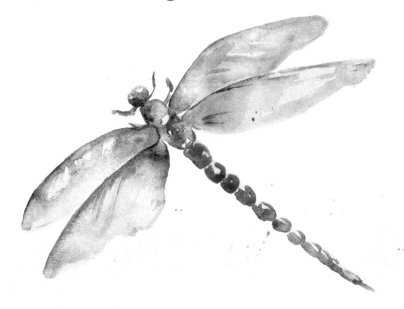

Your soul has unique talents and gifts available to help you move along your life path. Your talents are woven into your soul and are meant to enhance your gifts with action and expression of Divine love. I call the actions we take to use our talents while expressing God's love our "ings"—cooking, cleaning, painting, designing, creating, writing, running, snorkeling and so forth.

Your talents can aid you through your most challenging times by providing an outlet for your emotions and feelings to flow outward, while your gifts can comfort you by bringing the flow of Divine love inward, guiding and reassuring you to face your lessons with ease. Your gifts are the support system that connect you to the Divine.

Living your life's purpose is a scary feat, and it requires your superhero Soul Self to rise to the occasion. Your talents can aid you through your most challenging times by providing an outlet for your emotions and feelings to flow outward, while your gifts can comfort you by bringing the flow of Divine love inward, guiding and reassuring you to face your lessons with ease.

You utilize your talents for expressing God's love when you set your intention to do so. Talents are actions steps. Anything you do with the intention of sharing love will support and open your gifts.

Connecting with the things you enjoy doing will help you discover your talents. Write down all of your "ings" below.

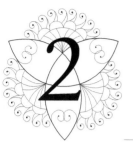

You can connect with the Divine through your gifts or as they are commonly known, your clairs. The easiest way to decipher Spirit's guidance is by being in tune with your senses. Use the lines below to write down your five senses; sight, smell, sound, taste, and feel. Describe in detail what you notice about each of your senses.

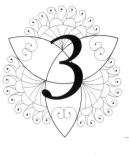

Being aware of your talents and gifts is important, but we must also focus on healing your blocks. If you try to just fix, outrun, cover or hide your pain, you will never find the relief your soul needs. Avoiding your pain and your healing leaves you feeling depleted and unhappy.

What is your pain trying to show you?

Believe... JOURNAL

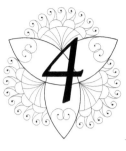

The subconscious triggers cause worry within you, which bring thoughts that arise and overshadow God's love for you. You end up denying the guidance from Spirit, mistrusting your gifts and turning off your connection.

What worries are overshadowing your Divine truth?

Believe... JOURNAL

CHAPTER EIGHT

PURE OF HEART

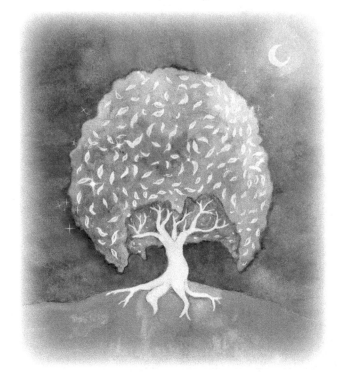

Y**ou are born with the gift of being your own healer through the connection to Spirit.** Your soul is energy sensitive and has come into life with the ability to channel love and heal your deepest wounds. This pure love is woven through your DNA and your energy centers and gives you the ability to channel Divine love.

The empath who is affected by earth-bound energy can feel and take on other beings' energy within their bodies. A sensitive soul who feels the earth-bound energy on the outside of their body is equally challenged by it. And the pure of heart, who can be either an empath or a sensitive soul, has an extrasensory ability to connect to Spirit and channel Divine love.

There are many aspects to being an empath or sensitive soul. When you come to terms with your gifts and how you can use them, you can utilize your energy for the greater good, for clear intuitive guidance, and/or for helping others. The goal is to have you moving and grooving in your energy in a healthy, high vibe state. Then you will experience the energy around you but will do so without taking it on as part of your being. Being a healthy empath or sensitive soul means you are able to decipher the different layers and tones of energy as you channel Divine love to others.

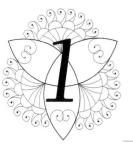

Invite the presence of an Angel to come forward.

Can you physically see an Angel in front of you? Describe how you see or sense this Angel.

Has God or a religious figure ever appeared to you?
Write about it.

Think of what it feels like when someone is angry with you. What do you notice about the energy around and inside your body?

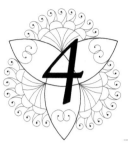

An empath is affected by earth-bound energy and can feel and take on other beings' energy within their bodies. Sensitive souls feel energy on the outside of their body.

How would you describe yourself and your relationship with energy?

CHAPTER NINE

WHAT GOD WANTS US TO KNOW

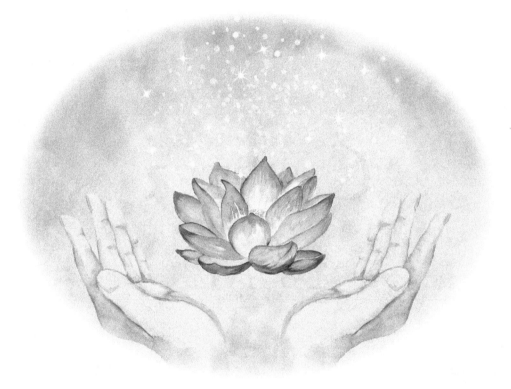

Love is always available to you. Divine Source wants you to remember that you are loved and that Holy Love lives within you. Your strength is bigger than you believe, and just because you are born, you are invaluable. You are all meant to be here, and you are perfect in the Divine's eyes! The Divine also wants you to know that forgiveness sets you free. You have been given this most awesome gift: A chance to be your best self and to set free those who have caused you pain.

God speaks to all life. You can turn on your receptors by opening your senses and your chakras to hear Him. God wants to hang out with you every day! Raising your energy through journaling will help you to meet the Divine, this is how you can connect with ease.

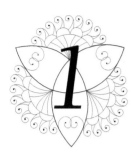

Separation from love happens for most during childhood, from the conditioning and belief systems of the adults in your life. This conditioning might teach you that you aren't smart, that you behave badly, are mean, are funny-looking or have big ears.

What did your early conditioning teach you?
What do you now understand that you could not as a child?

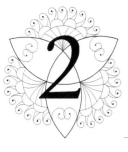

Do you often worry and stress about your preferred outcome instead of focusing on love and trusting Divine love?
Describe one instance wherein you did this, as well as the effect it had on the situation.

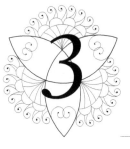

Repeat the healing mantra "I am the grace of God" three times while holding your hands palm over palm on your heart center. Inhale, filling your chest cavity with air, and slowly exhale.
Then, share your feelings and experience with this exercise.

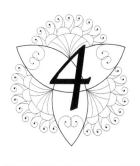

When you say "Amen" at the end of a prayer or mantra, it means you agree with the statement, and so it is. This aligns you with Divine truth and intention. Repeat these three life-changing truths: I am loved unconditionally. Amen. I am invaluable. Amen. Forgiveness sets me free. Amen.

Write down how you feel repeating these truths.

CHAPTER TEN

HOW CAN LOVE SUPPORT US?

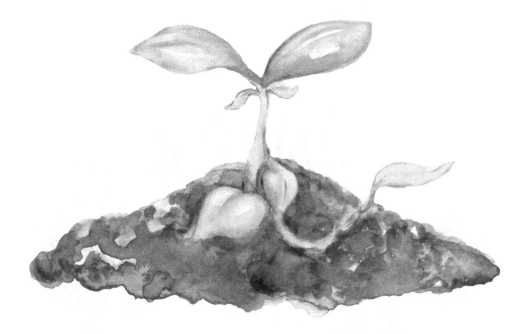

Love is so vast in energy that it is not easily confined by the walls of the mind. Like religions that teach within four walls and keep you contained under an umbrella of their belief system, you also have walls around your personal beliefs about love and God.

The vastness of love and God is within you. You are the foundational dwelling in which God, spirituality, love, compassion, faith, joy, and hope all reside. There is always room for expansion in your personal relationship with love and God. Expansive thinking leads you to your soul's wisdom. Wisdom is God's gift to all humanity.

You can tap into your higher consciousness through journaling.

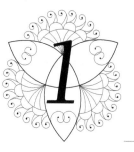

Love is always available to you. Think of a painful memory that you hold onto. Reflect with your Angels on how love was available to you. Share how you can release a layer of the old story and replace it with compassion on the lines below.

Pain is an indicator that something within you is out of balance. Do you live with pain? Share where your pain is located and how you can invite love into this area of your life.

Love supports you so you can heal one layer at a time. Write a letter to your pain or trauma and ask it how love can help you and what it needs to heal.

As you grow with love you find that loving another is easy but loving yourself is not always easy. You are meant to be here! Use the lines below to speak loving truths to yourself and how love supports you..

CHAPTER ELEVEN

Saints And Sinners

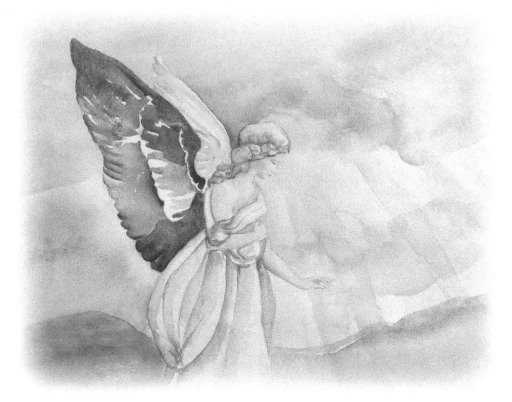

Saints are souls that have lived with the promises that love offers them, as well as to those they serve. They have been guided to serve humanity through various charitable actions. A saint is known as someone who was embodied to live in a state of holiness and to dedicate their life to Divine law.

Sinners are souls that live and have lived with the *fear* of love's promises. They are living beings who have committed an act that is against Divine law and God. Manifesting with God provides you with truthful insights. It brings clarity to the Divine timing at play. In return for the "you work" you do as you manifest, you heal and grow while you experience joy.

By participating as the saint of your own life, you actually get to be of service, heal and receive. Sainthood therefore is not out of your reach. A life of being in service, of walking within your soul's truths, is filled with moments that call you to serve with faith as your guidepost and receive abundance in Divine time.

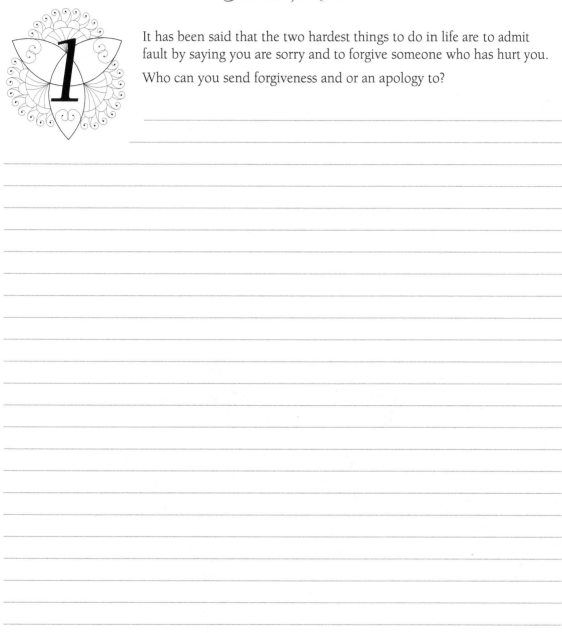

It has been said that the two hardest things to do in life are to admit fault by saying you are sorry and to forgive someone who has hurt you.

Who can you send forgiveness and or an apology to?

Place your right hand on your crown chakra on the top of your head and begin slowly tapping with your pointer finger as your internal eyesight focuses on the crown. With your intention, invite the flow of love energy to the crown chakra until you feel filled with love. Then, write down your experience.

With your eyes closed, focus on your third eye chakra in the center of your forehead. Allow any thoughts to simply pass by as you remain present in this moment.

Using your right middle finger, gently begin tapping slowly on your heart center. As the breath enters, it gently flows inward connecting and igniting love energy to flow.

Share your feelings and experience here.

You are love and are meant to share your light with others.
How do you feel called to serve others?

CHAPTER TWELVE

FROM THE "I" TO THE "WE"

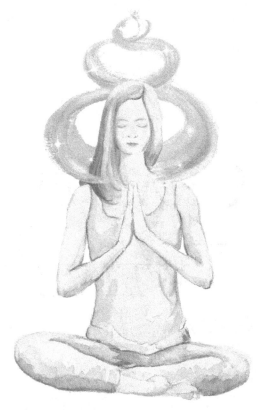

The "I" is the inner ego craving attention, and the "we" is the uniting of souls. When you focus on the "I," you can become isolated and feel alone. Those feelings spark emotions, and you end up questioning God.

Angels have taught me about energy; energy between people and situations look like threads of light, similar to a Twizzlers Pull 'n' Peel. These thin cords connect you to your life stories. While you may be unaware that these cords are there, you definitely can feel when your energy is being drained. In order to stop being depleted, you can disconnect from the energetic source that's depleting you. You can separate from the relationships that don't serve you. This allows you to heal the "we" by focusing on love for both points of view. This practice will help you to welcome new, loving, and, vibrant relationships into your life.

The Angels say that fear's grip is revealed when you are focused on serving the "I," which is your ego's needs, wants and desires.

List out your desires and notice which ones serve the "I" and which are in service to the greater good.

Bring your attention to the center of your chest. Feel your heart chakra begin to open with the most beautiful emerald-green light that pours all around your body.

Share how you feel, in writing, before moving on to the next prompt.

Within your heart chakra, begin to notice cords of energy. Take a moment to sense these cords and what they look like. Notice that while some of the cords look healthy and strong, others may look darker and less vibrant.

Write down a person or an event that has caused you pain. With a prayerful mind, bow in reverence to this energy while inviting your energy cord to disconnect before writing about your experience and moving to the next prompt.

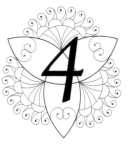

As you release their energy from you, your cord is released from them. It returns to a healthy state and is replaced in your heart. A sense of relief washes over you, and the energy of the past fades out of sight. Your body absorbs the love, and a renewal of energy takes place.

Write down how you feel at the completion of this exercise.

Chapter Thirteen

LOVE SPARK

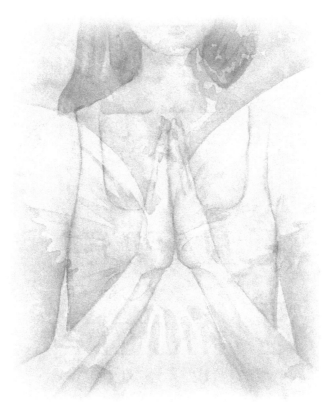

When you connect to the Divine truth that you are love, the miracle moments that are meant for you are welcomed in through your faith. You can practice your "you work" by showing up for yourself first, then for others.

We are living in a time that is in need of a great healing. It's time to heal your pain, your thoughts, and your actions. Love is needed to clean up your opinions. It is an era in which you are called to face your greatest fears and see beyond them to experience love fully. Love heals, while fear imprisons. When you make the choice to be the love, you can be of service and help humanity.

The gifts from the Divine are meant to help, guide, and support you through the good times, challenging times, and the times you fall from grace. The Angels will always provide you with love and assistance, you just need to invite them in!

Miracles are available to every soul. Yes, this means you!
Are you in need of a miracle? You need only ask!

Share what you need on the lines below.

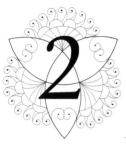

The Angels will always provide you with love and assistance, as long as you ask. Sharing your gratitude aligns you with a higher vibration, which helps facilitate this process.

Write your Angels a note of gratitude and petition.

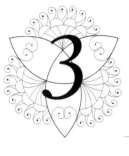

It's time to heal our collective pains, thoughts and actions. Love is needed to cleanup your opinions.

Write about how you can clean up your thoughts to help heal collective pain.

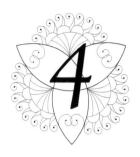

There are two universal truths that the Angels shared.

The first is that the soul is infinite, meaning you are here on Earth and with God at the same time. This also means that the separation you experience when a loved one dies is just of the physical body; the soul remains connected to you, always.

The second one is that we all want to be loved, equally. To express love, you must first love yourself then share that outward with others.

Write a love note to a departed loved one. Then, be still and feel them answer you back through your writing. Record their response with love and gratitude.

Believe... JOURNAL

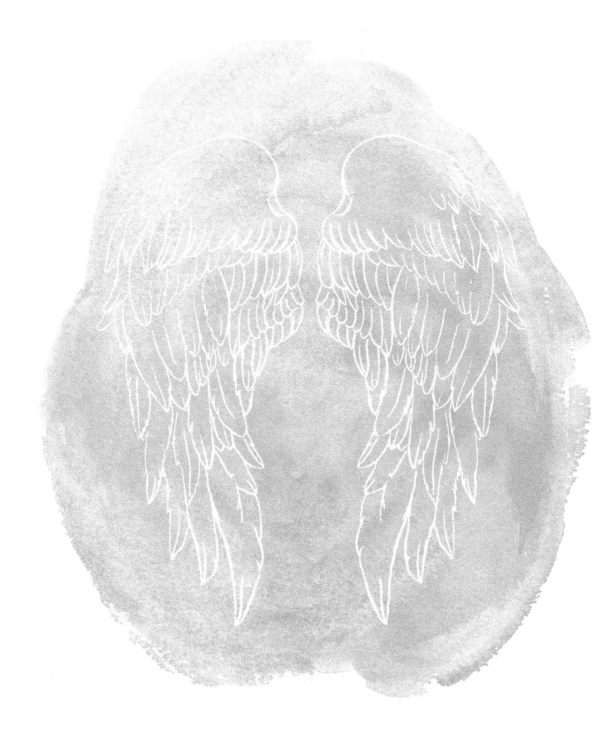

Congrats! I am so happy you have honored and loved yourself through this journal.

I know that you experienced many feelings and emotions during our time together. Despite this, you continued on. Your personal "you work" is your soul evolving closer to Divinity and your Holy self.

You can come back to these pages and prompts to deepen your connection to the Divine and to your soul-self. Every time you return to an exercise you will take off another layer, revealing new energy that helps you feel lighter and brighter about yourself.

May God's love be ever present within your being as you continue evolving on your soul's journey. Amen.

blessings Xx, *Jeanne*

About the Author

Internationally acclaimed spirital medium, healer, author and speaker, Jeanne Street, is a Catholic girl in an Angel world. She works with the Spiritual realm embodying the Holy Spirit while illuminating Divine compassion and love through her work.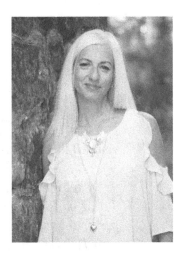

Jeanne was born into this life with the beautiful gift of connection. She has the ability to see, feel, hear and speak to both the departed and celestial beings.

Through her connection and clear knowing her sessions and readings are precise and detailed. Jeanne has helped thousands of individuals navigate through difficult events in their lives. Jeanne's deepest desire is to help people heal their pain and trauma.

Jeanne provides connection to Spirit, Angels and departed loved ones through private and small group readings, large group events, and through her books, **The Goddess You** and **The Goddess Journal, Believe . . . Angels Don't Lie** and **Angels Don't Lie, Believe . . .Journal**. She also offers Divine lifestyle products, accessories and a vast array of resources that are available on her website.

Jeanne's loving and accurate connections have transformed the lives of her private clients and public podcast listeners, as well as the live audience on her show **Angels Don't Lie**.

Jeanne resides in Connecticut with her devoted husband of 35 years, her 4 grown children, her daughter and son in law and 5 grandchildren and counting.

About the Illustrator

A life-long artist, Eileen has been an active graphic designer and illustrator since 1992.

Eileen was excited and inspired when Jeanne offered her the chance to apply her talents and help craft **Believe...Angels Don't Lie** and the accompanying **Angles Don't Lie, Believe... Journal**. For as long as she can remember, Eileen has loved taking part in the creative process, and engaging her superpower of identifying details others often overlook. This ability earned her the moniker 'Eagle Eye' from her dad at a young age.

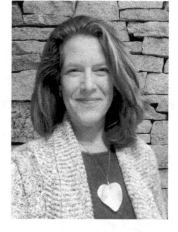

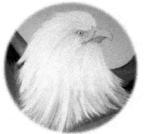

Children's wall mural painted by Eileen Portelance

A Catholic and deeply passionate woman, Eileen has been transformed by Jeanne Street's Angel world. The healing meditations, personal readings, life lessons and love she has experienced working alongside Jeanne and the team has allowed her to rediscover the joy in design and illustration once again. She looks forward to many more collaborations with Jeanne and the **Angels Don't Lie** community in the future.

Eileen has worked as a senior-level artist in new product development, marketing, and publishing, primarily in educational markets. Her work has earned her accolades such as the Teacher's Choice Award from Learning Magazine. She is a graduate of Western Connecticut State University in graphic design/illustration and is a certified art teacher. She loves contributing to community projects and is particularly proud of the 5th grade mural at Western CT Academy for International Studies in Danbury, CT that she helped orchestrate.

A Connecticut resident, Eileen can be found hiking the local hills and taking walks on sandy beaches with her husband since 1993, watching her three children and step-son transform into adults, and seeing the family dog, Griffin, act like a puppy from time to time.

You can find her portfolio and artistic interests at, *eileenportelance.com*

Spiritual support
for your soul's growth

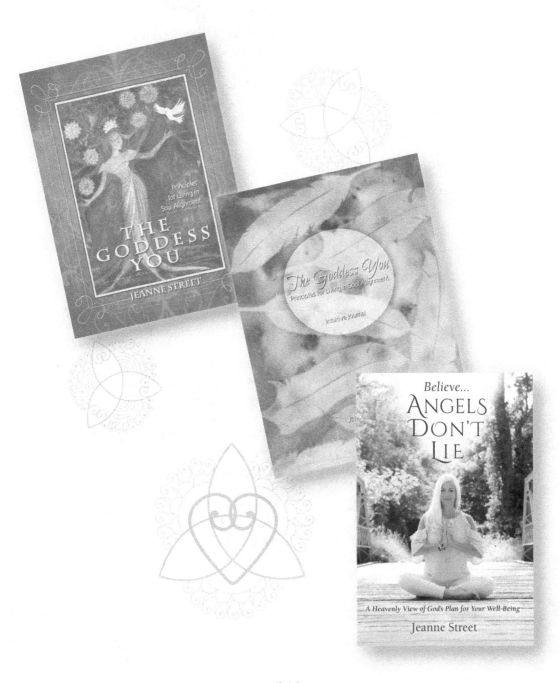

Continue to feel supported & spritually aligned EVERYDAY!

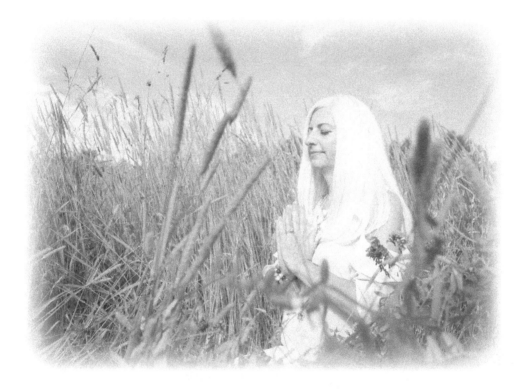

visit me at....

www.jeannestreet.com

https://www.facebook.com/Jeannestreetmedium/

https://www.instagram.com/jeannestreetmedium/

CPSIA information can be obtained
at www.ICGtesting.com
Printed in the USA
LVHW022031210820
663784LV00009B/509